Covid-

All Lies

All Crime

Facts and Figures

Paul M L Weston

About the Author

Paul Weston is a political commentator who writes about a variety of issues related to the ongoing battles between the centre-right and the "progressive" left. Covid-19 and all other medical industry realities were not on his radar prior to 2020 but became a matter of supreme importance when it rapidly became apparent that vaccines and health were being used to usher in a whole new way of controlled life for everyone on planet earth.

Every chapter of this book will be available to watch or read on my Rumble and Substack accounts, as will further output concerning the Covid-19 and the ensuing fall-out. The beauty of electronic media allows easy access to links, so I encourage people to watch/read via those sites if they wish to verify my sources via the simplicity of a mouse click.

https://substack.com/@paulweston

https://rumble.com/c/c-741735

https://www.youtube.com/@paulweston3663/videos

https://www.patreon.com/user?u=65319756&fan_landing=true

Contents

1: Introduction   9

2: Fraudulent Excess Deaths   13

3: Manufacturing Excess Deaths   19

4: The Great Care Home Cull   27

5: Matt Hancock's Role   33

6: Manipulating the Death Rate Data   41

7: Flu Deaths V Covid-19 Deaths in 2020   45

8: The PCR Fraud   51

9: How It Started   57

10: Lockdowns   61

11: Did Lockdowns & Masks Work?   65

12: Do I Need the Covid Vaccine?   71

13: Does it work?   73

14: Is It Safe?   77

15: The Pfizer Trial   85

16: Pfizer's Criminal Past   89

17: Is It Even a Vaccine?   93

18: Rewriting Medical Language   99

19: Afterword   101

20: References   105

Chapter 1: Introduction

Could our political masters push another health emergency on the world again, with all the attendant losses of liberty? I believe so, yes. The World Health Organisation (WHO) is actively engaged in pursuing new powers which will give them near total control over our governments should a new "pandemic" materialise. WHO Director General, Tedros Adhanom Ghebreyesus, has repeatedly stated this is a question of when, rather than if.

Bill Gates is of the same view. He has smirkingly stated "the next one (pandemic) will really get their attention". Gates is a massive investor in the vaccine industry, of course. He also gives vast amounts of money to the WHO and exercises a great deal of control over Tedros Adhanom Ghebreyesus, a man essentially engineered into his position of power by Bill Gates himself.

"Power" is the word best associated with the entire Covid-19 pandemic. Second best would be "billionaire". Whilst the little people (by which I mean you and I) were herded, terrorised, manipulated and coerced into obeying our masters, the billionaire class amassed yet more wealth whilst the political class amassed huge new levels of control over their citizens.

This power grab was planned down to the last detail. In October 2019, the World Economic Forum (WEF) along with Johns Hopkins University and The Bill & Melinda Gates Foundation, co-hosted an extraordinary meeting called Event 201, which detailed proposed plans of action in the event of a lethal, global pandemic.

Less than six-months later these plans were put into action across the planet. All tried and trusted historical responses to viral epidemics were abandoned in favour of lockdowns, masks, and social distancing. Our immune systems were considered redundant. Quarantining the healthy, until a miracle potion invented by the pharmaceutical industry could save mankind, became the order of the day.

 A few basic questions need to be asked about the entire Covid-19 pandemic:

1) Was the Covid-19 virus as lethal as we were told?

2) Were lockdowns, masks & social distancing an appropriate response?

3) Did we really need the vaccine?

4) Does the vaccine actually work?

5) Is the vaccine safe?

6) Is the mRNA vaccine even a vaccine?

7) Were the vaccine trials conducted ethically, honestly, and impartially?

8) Can we trust our Health Regulation Agencies?

9) Did our governments ever have our best interests at heart?

10) Or were/are they instead, promoting a tyrannical Globalist Agenda?

If the answers to these questions are all "no" (save question 10) then further questions need to be asked. Such as: what on earth happened to the world after March 2020? Who drove it? Why did they do so? What does it mean with regard to our future in terms of freedom or tyranny?

The very first issue that needs to be addressed is the death rate seen across the world in 2020. We were told Covid-19 was a lethal virus that could kill millions of people globally. We were told this presented the greatest peacetime threat the world had seen in recent history.

Was this true?

Chapter 2. Fraudulent Excess Deaths

One simple graph reveals a great deal about the supposed vast numbers of Covid-19 deaths in 2020. This graph is related to the UK but is typical of most Western countries. It shows the number of deaths per 100,000 people (which takes into account a growing or declining population) between 1942-2020.

Source of graph[1] : <u>Office For National Statistics - Annual deaths and mortality rates 1838 to 2020</u>

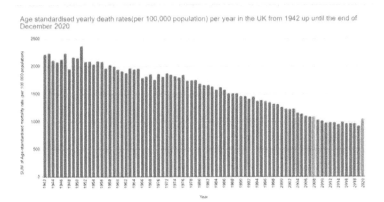

Age standardised yearly death rates(per 100,000 population) per year in the UK from 1942 up until the end of December 2020

As you can see, the death rate in the UK in 2020 was much the same as 2008 (the two orange bars) and lower than every year between 1942 to 2007. In what possible way then, can this possibly be termed a lethal pandemic?

As I say, the UK was little different in terms of overall deaths when compared to the rest of the world. This can easily be confirmed by looking at figures for the global population.

In 2019 the global population numbered approximately 7.76 billion. In 2020 approximately 7.84 billion. In 2021 approximately 7.9 billion. In 2022 approximately 7.98 billion. 2020 saw a broadly similar rise in global population growth as the other years. This would be an impossibility had there really been a lethal pandemic stalking the land in 2020 – as we were repeatedly told.

People are born, they hopefully live a good long life and then they die. To state the obvious, this is completely natural and normal. Approximately 1% of a Western country's population die every year. The vast majority of these deaths are amongst the very old and the very ill. In a bad flu year, the annual death rate might rise from 1% to 1.1%. In a good year it might drop from 1% to 0.9%.

Between the years 2000 to 2019, approximately 1.1% of the UK population died. As is completely normal. The average age of those who died during those years was eighty-one. The average number of life-threatening illnesses they suffered from was three-point-five and were, in the main, heart disease, diabetes, high blood pressure, kidney failure etc.

In 2020, the year of the Covid-19 pandemic, approximately 1% of the population died. As is completely normal. The average age of death was eighty-two. The average number of life-threatening illnesses they suffered from was three-point-five and were, in the main, heart disease, diabetes, high blood pressure, kidney failure etc.

To reiterate then, between 2000-2019 an average 1.1% of the population died every year. The overwhelming majority were very old and very ill. In 2020, the year of the "killer pandemic" 1% of the population died. The overwhelming majority were very old and very ill.

How strange. How inexplicably strange. Pandemic Year 2020 actually saw a slight decrease in overall death percentages compared to the two previous decades. This isn't my opinion; it is a verifiable fact. This isn't a computer modelled data set; it is a verifiable and historical fact.

In short, there was no lethal pandemic in 2020. Yet nearly all the Western governments locked us down after declaring a Public Health Emergency. They scared us silly every day with terror-porn about gazillions of excess deaths. This makes no sense at all. It was all a lie. One can only conclude there was an alternative agenda at play.

Most people tend not realise just how many people die every day from old age/natural causes. The perfectly natural and normal 1% death rate in

England, a country of 56 million people, equates to 560,000 deaths annually or 1,500 daily. In America, a country of 330 million, the 1% death rate equates to 3.3 million annually or 9,000 daily.

I mention this only to show how easy it is for corrupt governments and media outlets to take advantage of such huge numbers. All they need do is attach the label of "Covid-19 Death" to a percentage of perfectly natural and normal deaths in order to shriek a headline of "Last Week Saw Three Thousand Deaths From Covid-19!" emblazoned above a bar-chart of death coloured Red! Red! Danger Red! Which is exactly what our corrupt governments and MSM outlets did.

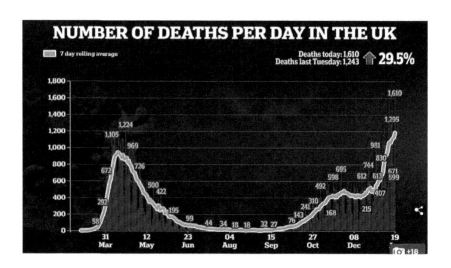

16

That said, a sizeable number of above average excess deaths was a necessary precondition in March and April 2020 to both shock the newly locked down population into fearful submission, and to crush any questions from the MSM about the genuine seriousness of the pandemic – not that many MSM journalists had the slightest interest.

How did our politicians find a shockingly large and wonderfully convenient number of excess deaths over a short time frame in order to kick-start the pandemic? That was easy. They simply engineered them in a war against the old and the ill - and thus already close to death - in our Care Homes.

Chapter 3: Manufacturing Excess Deaths

Why did Western governments portray Covid-19 as something resembling the 14th Century Black Death, which killed close to 50% of the European population? If we are to be brutally honest, we must ask whether a government capable of deliberately misrepresenting the death rate figures could actually be capable of engineering real deaths, actual deaths, in order to drive their peculiar agenda. Could they really do that?

The answer to that is yes. Not all Western governments, admittedly, but the two most guilty of doing so were America and Great Britain, which immediately after declaring a public health emergency and locking us down, initiated an inexplicable policy with regard to the elderly and the ill which at best could be described as criminal incompetence, and at worst, mass murder. The following graph effectively sums up what happened in 2020:

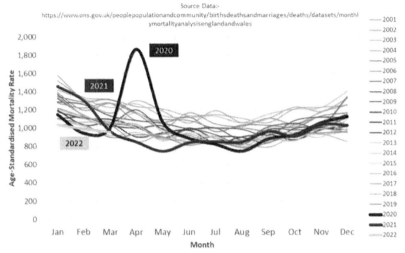

Monthly Age-Standardised Mortality Rate Per 100K Population
Deaths Registered in England
2001 to 2022

Source Data:-
https://www.ons.gov.uk/peoplepopulationandcommunity/birthsdeathsandmarriages/deaths/datasets/monthlymortalityanalysisenglandandwales

The graph is sourced[1] from The Office for National Statistics website. It tracks total monthly death figures in England and Wales for every year between 2001 and 2022. Each year is represented by a different colour. 2020 is dark blue.

As we can see, between the beginning of January and the middle of March 2020, the death rate was lower than the nineteen preceding years. Deaths start to rise stratospherically in mid-March, before peaking in mid-April and subsequently dropping below and staying below the nineteen-year average from mid-May to the end of the year.

20

If we divide the year of 2020 into four quarters, we see well below average deaths in Q1 and Q3. Average deaths in Q4, and a huge bulge over a six-week period of Q2. How can this be explained?

Before I get onto that, it should be noted this Q2 bulge in excess deaths did not happen in all Western countries. Of the countries where it did happen, Britain and America (principally New York) were the two glaring examples. Obtaining data from America's Centers for Disease Control and Prevention (CDC) is notoriously complicated, if not deliberately impossible. Hence my use of data from Britain's Office for National Statistics.

As we now know, all Western governments more or less acted in lockstep during 2020. Mid-March saw the implementation of what was initially touted as just two-or-three-week lockdowns. From the moment they started, Britain and America thought it a terrifically good idea to immediately move old and ill people from hospitals - without testing them for Covid-19 — into Care Homes.

The reasoning behind this, or so they tell us, was to free-up hospital space for the gazillions of Covid patients predicted by Bill Gates funded computer modellers to shortly overwhelm every hospital in the West. In reality, the hospitals were far emptier in 2020 than they had been for decades.

Having pump-primed American and English care homes with Covid-19, they were promptly declared off-limits to relatives (who were all locked down anyway) and remained that way for more than a year. Worse still, doctors self-declared the care homes off-limits to doctors as well, whilst the government advised care home managers that ill residents who showed signs of Covid-19 should be quarantined and effectively treated as End-of-Life patients.

On top of all these ingredients for a mass culling of the elderly, Do Not Resuscitate Notices (DNR's) were illegally blanket issued without the knowledge of the care home residents' families. As far as I am aware, no one has yet swung for this terrible crime.

Covid-19 symptoms are not dissimilar to the common cold or influenza, and as care home staff had been terrified into believing they would probably die if they came into contact with Covid-19, the inevitable happened.

Perfectly healthy oldies with a sniffle were locked away in their rooms and treated as End-of-Life patients. Deprived of food and water they died in their tens-of-thousands between mid-March to the beginning of May 2020.

Think about this for a moment. Think about the behaviour of care home staff during 2020. It is not something covered by government experts and computer modellers, but it was perfectly natural behaviour when one considers the circumstances care home workers found themselves in.

By March 2020 we had been assured by our governments that Covid-19 was lethal. Videos were released via the mainstream media (MSM) of perfectly healthy Chinese chaps happily wandering through the streets of Wuhan before suddenly and ham-theatrically keeling over, twitching a bit, and then dying.

They were immediately scooped up by other Chinese chaps in bright orange Nuclear and Biological Warfare suits – who just happened to be passing by – all filmed by a civic-minded Chinese chappy who handed his video footage to the nearest Chinese Communist Party (CCP) chappy, who in turn passed it on to the unquestioning CNN and BBC.

Try then, to imagine being a care home worker in April 2020. Unable to recognise clumsily obvious terror-porn propaganda, and primed by the government to genuinely believe they could die if they contracted Covid-19, they were told on Monday that their care home would be taking in a number of ill and untested patients from the local hospital on Wednesday.

Who in their right mind is going to risk death for a minimum wage return? Particularly so when care home workers believed the only reason potential

Covid-19 patients were being foisted upon them was because the higher paid hospital doctors and nurses (all equally terrified of dying from Covid-19) simply wanted them as far away from their hospitals as possible. Which was of course, very much the case.

So, terrified care home workers; blanket (and illegal) DNR notices; no visiting relatives to explain anything to; no emotional bond whatsoever with the newly arrived - and possibly deadly disease carrying - defenceless elderly; no visiting doctors to explain anything to; government and local GP Surgery advice to treat fit and healthy residents with cold/flu symptoms as End-of-Life Covid-19 patients. Result? The Great Care Home Cull. All absolutely inevitable, given the circumstances.

The greatest tragedy (or crime) in American and British Care Homes was that regardless of the existence or non-existence of a lethal respiratory virus called Covid-19, the elderly residents of the care homes were consigned to die anyway as the direct and inevitable consequence of government policies.

Many died from loneliness. Relatively fit and physically healthy residents suffering from dementia could not understand why their sons, daughters and grandchildren had abandoned them. In their misery, they just gave up. They had nothing to look forward to. Indeed, many thought their children suddenly hated them and no longer wanted to see them. And so they died. Lonely, confused and heartbroken.

Those who became moderately but survivably ill from a heavy cold or the flu were simply barricaded in their rooms by terrified care home staff. They too died lonely, heartbroken and confused, just like the dementia sufferers. But it was even worse for the flu symptom residents. They died from starvation and dehydration as well. What happened in our care homes was truly a Crime Against Humanity.

Chapter 4: The Great Care Home Cull

If we can agree that a huge death toll was pretty much the inevitable consequence of government action in American and British Care Homes, it forces us into asking a number of questions. The first of which must be: was it deliberately and cold-bloodedly planned, or was it simply the result of government incompetence?

At the very outset of the Covid-19 emergency, Britain's dead-eyed Chief Medical Officer, Chris Whitty, stated the Covid-19 virus was relatively innocuous for the young, the fit and the healthy, and only presented a risk of death to the very old and the very ill.

Matt Hancock, the British Health Secretary at the time, stated he would throw a "ring of steel" around Britain's Care Homes. In a manner of speaking, he did just that, but only insofar as making it impossible for relatives of care home residents to breach the ring of steel in order to visit their aged, loved ones.

Imagine the surreal levels of incompetence necessary to inadvertently slaughter tens-of-thousands of old and ill elderly residents of care homes, having implicitly stated only the old and ill were vulnerable, and that wherever they were, a defensive "ring of steel" would be erected around them.

It is very hard to believe it was simply a matter of incompetence. There are a number of issues which reinforce this belief. If you cast your mind back to April and May 2020, what was being shown 24/7 on the TV news and in the newspapers? What were we being told 24/7 by our politicians?

Answer: We were in the grip of a deadly pandemic. Thousands were dying. Hospitals were swamped with Covid-19 patients. Exhausted doctors and nurses were working around the clock "on the front lines" in the war against Covid. We were *all* vulnerable. We must stay at home. This message was hammered home for the entirety of 2020.

Were the hospitals swamped? Were thousands dying in our overwhelmed hospitals? The following graph suggest they were not.

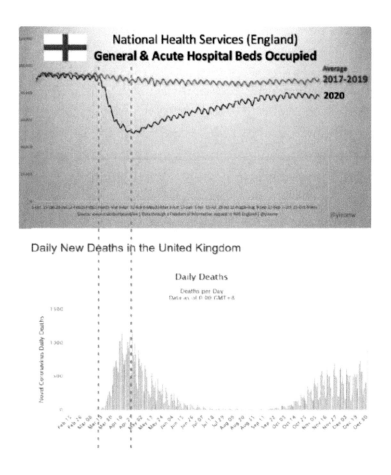

National Health Services (England)
General & Acute Hospital Beds Occupied

Average
2017-2019

2020

Daily New Deaths in the United Kingdom

Daily Deaths

Deaths per Day
Data as of 0.00 GMT +8

As you can clearly see, acute and general bed
occupancy plummeted in our hospitals during April
and May 2020, even as the daily Covid-19 deaths
reached hundreds and then thousands. So no, our
hospitals were not overwhelmed. If our doctors and
nurses were exhausted, it was only because so many
of them are so fat and so unfit they were unable to
keep up with the TikTok choreographer's dance

routine demands. If you think I am joking, just Google "Dancing Nurses" and weep.

Anyone who visited a hospital in post March 2020 knows they were virtually empty. Of course they were. All routine operations were cancelled. The only people "dying from Covid-19" in April and May 2020 were dying in the care homes, not the hospitals. And they were dying from loneliness, starvation and dehydration, not Covid-19.

I know several doctors and nurses. 2020 was a glorious holiday for them. Their gardens bloomed; their cars were shined and fettled; their bookshelves were built-in. And I will tell you something else: by June/July 2020 every single doctor told me the whole Covid-19 pandemic was a fraud of colossal proportions. Shamefully though, not one of them was prepared to say so publicly.

So, whilst doctors privately admitted the Great Covid Con, the news outlets prominently displayed continually updated death toll tickers on their sites. The daily headlines above lurid red (danger, danger!) graphs shrieked "Yet More Hundreds Dead Yesterday!" and "Covid-19 Death Toll Reaches New Record High!" All of this was lies. Outright, blatant lies.

We were never told the only excess deaths occurred over just a six-week period, and only in the Care Homes. Instead, we were told large numbers of excess deaths from Covid-19 continued to occur in our overloaded hospitals throughout the year. None of this was true. It was all lies.

We were never told those dying were **only** amongst the very old and very ill. Instead, we were told people of all ages were dying, even the young and healthy. None of this was true. It was all lies.

We were never told that death rates were average or below average between June 2020 and January 2021. Instead, we were told there were thousands of Covid deaths occurring every week between those dates. None of this was true. It was all lies.

Chapter 5: Matt Hancock's Role

Ex-Health Secretary Matt Hancock suffers from dyslexia. He has trouble with words and numbers. Two words he should get very used to spelling and recognising are *geronticide* and *democide*. The former means the killing of the elderly. The latter, according to the Collins English Dictionary, means:

"The killing of members of a country's civilian population as a result of its government's policy, including by direct action, indifference, and neglect."

Hancock clearly suffers from a narcissistic personality disorder. He is also firmly aligned with Klaus Schwab and the World Economic Forum. In his tenure as British Health Secretary he was involved in various dubious instances where personal friends were awarded large government contracts for Covid-19 related procurements. And, of course, whilst he was telling us to lockdown and avoid all personal contact with others, he was carrying out an adulterous and very up-close and personal liaison with his squeeze Gina Coladangelo.

In the furore following the Coladangelo affair, Hancock was pushed out of the government's inner circle and sought to rebuild his career by appearing on trash TV reality shows. Never has there been a man so unsuited to run a whelk stall, let alone oversee the government's reaction to an allegedly unprecedented emergency.

Or at least "so unsuited" in normal times. 2020 was far from normal however, so perhaps Hancock was engineered into his position as Health Secretary precisely because of his callous and cold-hearted inabilities, rather than despite them. After all, it takes a particularly wicked sort of human-being to do the dirty work sometimes required by those who set the Globalist Agenda. Hancock was an absolute Godsend to those in need of immediate and large numbers of deaths.

In late 2020, *Amnesty International* issued a 54-page report[1] into the Great Care Home Cull. *Amnesty* didn't go quite so far as to unequivocally state it was an exercise in mass murder, but it got very close to doing so by implication. *Amnesty* also called for a full government inquiry. To date, this has not happened. Nor has The Great Care Home Cull been forensically dissected in the ongoing governmental inquiry into the pandemic. In point of fact, both it and the *Amnesty* Report have been disappeared, vapourised, or Memory-Holed as Orwell might have put it.

Hancock is aware he is in some danger of prosecution for Democide. He has already stated he believes government officials should be indemnified against prosecution for deaths resulting from ministerial action taken during an international emergency. The problem he faces is that the deaths were caused only by government action as opposed to a viral pandemic.

Hancock was videotaped[2] on April 17th 2020, casually informing his interlocutor, one Dr Luke Evans, that he had stockpiled a sufficient amount of Midazolam - a drug used to slowly shut down the respiratory system, which when coupled with morphine painlessly eases those at end-of-life over the finishing line.

As it turns out, Hancock managed to obtain a two-year supply of Midazolam. Or a two-year supply in normal times. In abnormal 2020 there was no danger of it exceeding its sell-by date. Between March and June, large amounts were used up. Lots and lots of Midazolam, coupled with tens-of-thousands of deaths at the precise same time in the Care Homes we were not allowed to enter. See the following graphs:

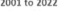

Monthly Age-Standardised Mortality Rate Per 100K Population
Deaths Registered in England
2001 to 2022

Source Data:-
https://www.ons.gov.uk/peoplepopulationandcommunity/birthsdeathsandmarriages/deaths/datasets/monthl
ymortalityanalysisenglandandwales

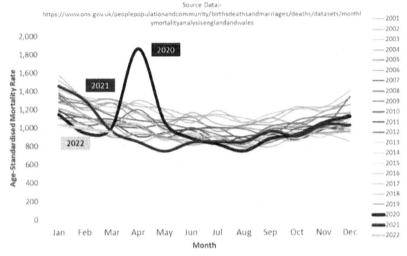

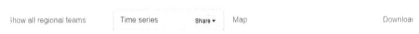

Items for Midazolam hydrochloride + Midazolam hydrochloride + Midazolam maleate ...
by all regional teams

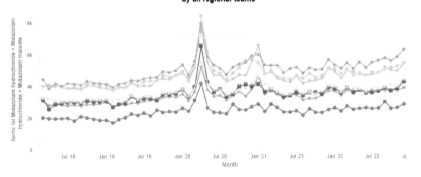

In a 2023 court case, Hancock claimed he had never heard of Midazolam before being accused of using it to murder care home residents. He lied. He committed perjury. He is on tape talking about it three years earlier. Hancock then went on to post a message on his TikTok account (why, WHY does an ex-Minister of State have a TikTok account?) aimed at those who accused him of The Midazolam Murders, in which he demonically laughed and said[3]: "Ha-ha- ha, oh no, I'm devastated, ha-ha-ha".

This TikTok video outburst is extraordinary. I'm not a psychiatrist, but Hancock seems to be exhibiting a real degree of psychopathology here. We know from a *Daily Telegraph* article[4] that Hancock's NHS was instructed to deny care to the elderly in care homes. We know the National Institute for Health and Care Excellence (NICE) published their ng163 Guidance[5] on April 3rd, 2020, advising Midazolam to be issued to patients who exhibited "anxiety" and breathlessness. Needless to say, prescribing Midazolam to people struggling to breathe is nothing other than a death sentence.

NICE actually stated the following: "Sedation and opioid use should not be withheld because of a fear of causing respiratory depression" and went on to say: "Notes: At the time of publication (April 2020), opioids and benzodiazepines did not have a UK marketing authorisation for this indication or route of administration…"

In another video, Hancock was asked about the Do Not Resuscitate (DNR) notices issued in care homes without the knowledge of the resident's families. He appeared as a rabbit in the headlights. Stuttering, stammering, squirming, he guiltily said this:

"I totally agree with you about the, er, the, the, er, the inexcusable, erm, nature of any attempt to use Do Not Resuscitate orders without consent, and when, erm, there were concerns raised at blanket consent being put in place, erm, we stopped that immediately".

We stopped that immediately, said Hancock. But too late, of course, to stop the deaths. Which one can only assume was all part of the plan. A question not asked was just who issued the blanket DNR orders in the first place. It wouldn't have been Mrs Scroggins, the Care Home manageress, would it? Nor would it have been the local GP. The only person with the power to order such a wicked and murderously criminal action on a nationwide level could only have been Hancock himself.

Before I conclude this piece, let us look again at the dictionary definition of Democide: *"The killing of members of a country's civilian population as a result of its government's policy, including by direct action, indifference, and neglect".*

Conclusion: Did Health Secretary Matt Hancock deliberately put into place the mechanisms designed to ensure large numbers of deaths over a short space of time? Was this done in order to give some credibility to a claimed lethal pandemic which necessitated lockdowns and more? Did he engage in the colossal crime of Democide? Personally, I believe he did just that. And my belief is based purely on historical reality.

Footnote: The ng163 guidance disappeared from the NICE website but was retrieved courtesy of the miraculous internet archive *Wayback Machine*[6]

Chapter 6: Manipulating the Death Rate Data

If you have studiously ploughed through all the facts and figures so far, you must be wondering how on earth Western governments got away with the colossal fraud entailed in persuading us that Covid-19 deaths were enormously high throughout 2020. Ditto, that we were all equally threatened with death if we disobeyed the various ludicrous and tyrannical edicts crashing down upon us from the political, media, scientific and medical establishments.

What they did was actually very simple. Beautifully simple, in fact. They just applied the label of "Covid-19 death" to perfectly natural and normal deaths of the old and the ill, along with the deaths by terminally unfortunate accident of the young and the healthy.

Before PCR Testing became the norm, doctors were advised – without the actual necessity of looking at the recently departed – to label the death as a Covid-19 death if the deceased had shown any symptoms of Covid-19 such as breathlessness, fever, cough, cold etc. Needless to say, most old and ill people who die exhibit many of those symptoms.

After the PCR Testing regime became the norm, all deaths were labelled as Covid-19 if the deceased had tested PCR Positive. This included those who were dying from cancer, heart disease, stage-4 kidney disease etc. Mr X actually died of cancer, but Covid-19 was the label attributed to his death, simply because he had tested PCR positive two months earlier.

Even worse, a perfectly healthy twenty-one-year-old who died in a motorcycle accident was labelled a Covid-19 death if he had tested PCR positive three months previously. The government took some stick over this obviously fraudulent manipulation of mortality data, and decided to become less fraudulently insane by stating the PCR Positive Test must have taken place within twenty-eight days of the death.

This lessened the distortion to a degree, but nonetheless a fit and healthy twenty-five-year-old who died in a para-gliding accident was still labelled a Covid-19 death if he had tested positive at any point over the twenty-eight days between PCR test and para-glider plummet. All of this was criminally fraudulent, obviously, but it laid the groundwork for even more criminal insanity with regard to the future vaccines.

I don't want to get into the whole vaccine issue in this article but bear the following in mind: Fit and healthy thirty-year-old Mr Y was injected with the mRNA vaccine on Jan 1st, 2022. A few days later he felt a bit iffy and toddled along for a PCR test on January 5th which returned a positive result. On January 13th,

2022, poor old Mr Y suffered a heart attack whilst cycling and was pronounced dead at the scene.

The cause of death was listed as Covid-19. His family protested and said he had been feeling perfectly OK up to the date of the mRNA vaccine injection. Could the vaccine be responsible for his death, they asked the doctor. Of course not, she scoffed. Mr Y was technically unvaccinated, you see.

How is this possible? Western governments decreed it takes some days for mRNA vaccines to work – for them to be effective. So, a fourteen-day duration was put in place to allow for the delayed efficiency and/or nasty side effects following vaccination. If a person died thirteen days post vaccination, he/she was deemed technically unvaccinated.

Had they tested PCR positive within twenty-eight days from PCR positive test to heart attack whilst cycling however, they died from Covid-19. Even if they had been mRNA vaccinated within the exact same time frame.

Worse still, Mr Y will not only be fraudulently labelled as a Covid-19 death; he will also enter the government's statistical database as being unvaccinated, even though the vaccine may well have killed him. In turn, the government and the health agencies will use his "unvaccinated" death to encourage people to take the vaccine against Covid-19 death……

So simple. So wicked. So criminal. So obvious once your eyes are opened to the fraud.

Chapter 7: Flu Deaths V Covid-19 Deaths in 2020

According to the World Health Organisation (WHO), flu mysteriously disappeared[1] from the world in 2020. Actually, not quite all of 2020; it disappeared immediately after the Western governments initiated the Covid-19 lockdowns in March.

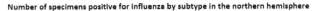

Number of specimens positive for influenza by subtype in the northern hemisphere

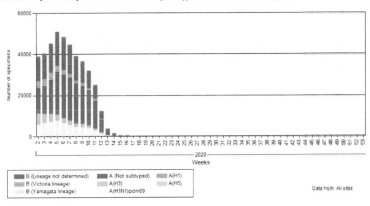

That is quite strange, isn't it? Almost as though all the usual respiratory deaths caused by flu in every year other than 2020 were simply re-labelled as Covid-19 related respiratory deaths in 2020. An easy way of finding out if this was the case is to look at the Office for National Statistics respiratory death data for 2019 and 2020.

In 2019 there were $71,674^2$ respiratory deaths. In 2020 there were $63,131^3$ respiratory deaths. This is rather strange too, considering the full name for Covid-19 is *Severe Acute **Respiratory** Syndrome Coronavirus 2.* I say strange, because it is most unusual – putting it mildly - to have a lower level of respiratory deaths during a supposedly apocalyptic pandemic driven by a virus which causes respiratory disease, no?

A death from influenza is medically the exact same as a death from Covid-19. It is a respiratory disease death. People die from an inability to breathe due to their lungs becoming congested with fluid, mucous, pus and blood. In reality, they die from viral pneumonia.

Influenza and Covid-19 cause pneumonia. No-one dies directly from the flu or Covid-19; they die from the viral pneumonia caused by Covid-19 and influenza - the symptoms of which are exactly the same from initial infection all the way through to pneumonia and possible death:

Stage 1: Cough/cold, feeling of heaviness in the chest, loss of appetite, fatigue.

Stage 2: Increase in cough intensity, shortness of breath, muscle aches, extreme fatigue, headaches, fever, chills, sweating, blue lips or nails due to lower blood oxygen levels.

Stage 3: Viral pneumonia, possible death.

The immune systems of healthy people can easily deal with flu or Covid-19 infections. You might feel terrible for a few days, but you soon get over it. Sadly, people with pre-existing serious illnesses (mostly old, but sometimes young) don't have very good immune systems. Hence the large numbers who die in a bad flu year.

To sum up the above then, influenza and Covid-19 both share the same symptoms, and both can lead to viral pneumonia and potential death. Especially so if left untreated. Is one more deadly than the other though? Studying the Infection Fatality Rates for both diseases provide an answer to that question.

The Infection Fatality Rate (IFR) expresses in percentage form the number of people who die after being infected by a particular disease.

The IFR for influenza varies between 0.1% and 0.2% depending upon a good year or a bad year for flu. This equates to 1 death for every 1,000 people infected in a good year, and 2 deaths per 1,000 people infected in a bad year.

According[4] to Cambridge University's MRC Biostatistics Unit, the IFR for Covid-19 between April 2020 and November 2021 was 0.25% which is essentially an extremely bad year for flu. The original MRC Biostatistics Unit study is curiously no longer available on their site, but fortunately I saved it in Dec 2021 on the ingenious Wayback Machine Internet Archive site, from where I was able to grab the graph below.

Epidemic summary

Current R_t	Number of infections	Attack rate	Current IFR	Change in infections incidence	Change in deaths incidence

Show 10 ∨ entries   Search: [   ]

	Age	Median	95% Crl (lower)	95% Crl (upper)
1	Overall	0.25%	0.25%	0.26%
2	<1yr,1-4	0.00083%	0.00026%	0.001%
3	5-14	0.00089%	0.00073%	0.0013%
4	15-24	0.0036%	0.0032%	0.0043%
5	25-44	0.023%	0.021%	0.026%
6	45-64	0.19%	0.18%	0.2%
7	65-74	0.83%	0.78%	0.88%
8	75+	3.2%	3.1%	3.4%

Showing 1 to 8 of 8 entries   Previous 1 Next

It is a little hard to read, so I will re-write it below. The Covid-19 IFR statistics are as follows:

Age 1-4:   0.00083%

Age 5-14:   0.00089%

Age 15-24:   0.0036%

Age 25-44:   0.23%

Age 45-64:   0.19%

Age 65-74:   0.83%

Age 75 Plus: 3.2%

The IFR for Covid-19 is an average of the seven sets of percentage figures above. It is heavily skewed by the 3.2% amongst those aged seventy-five and over. But even when this group is included, the IFR is still only 0.25% which is, as I say, not so very different from a particularly bad year for flu.

But we must bear something in mind here; most of the seventy-five-year-olds and over who died in 2020 were victims of the Great Care Home Cull. They didn't actually die from Covid-19 at all. They were effectively euthanised, yet their fraudulent Covid-19 death statistics play a hugely important part in skewing the IFR figures. If we disregard the seventy-five+ age group, the IFR drops to 0.17% which is pretty much in line with influenza.

As we can see, Covid-19 presented no more threat of death than the flu to those aged between one to seventy-five. In point of fact, there is a greater risk to the young in falling over and breaking their necks whilst making a catastrophically useless attempt at donning a pair of trousers than dying from Covid-19.

Conclusion: Influenza and Covid-19 have a similar Infection Fatality Rate and similar symptoms. Both cause respiratory death via pneumonia. Respiratory deaths were broadly similar in 2020 and 2019.

Somewhat mysteriously they were slightly lower in the year of the pandemic. Influenza miraculously disappeared in 2020. Could such an unprecedented event (or non-event) be even remotely possible? Of course not. Flu deaths were simply re-labelled as Covid-19 deaths. Genius.

Chapter 8: The PCR Fraud.

After the deaths driven by the Great Care Home Cull in Spring 2020 fizzled out, the government switched to positive PCR tests to drive the Covid Pandemic. These tests were dishonest and fraudulent.

According to the government's own research[1] the average range of false positive test results was 2.3% - which means out of 100,000 tests carried out, 2,300 (2.3% of 100,000) were false (caused by poor testing, storage, dirty instruments etc) and thus should be removed from the data.

If 100,000 tests returned 10,000 positive results, the **true** positive number would be 7,700 (10,000 positive tests minus 2,300 false positives).

If 100,000 tests returned 2,301 positive results, the true positive is only 1.

If 100,000 tests returned 2,300 positive results, the true positive is zero.

If 100,000 tests returned 2,999 positive results the true positive is minus 1, or in real life data, zero. All minus numbers are effectively zero, no matter how large or small.

Let us look at a typical day in 2020 then. According[2] to the government, 100,664 PCR tests were carried out on 31 May 2020, which returned 1,570 positive results.

For ease of argument, let us call the total number of tests carried out to be exactly 100,000 rather than 100,664.

So, 100,000 tests returned 1,570 positive results. The government claimed 1,570 new Covid-19 cases that day, because they didn't deduct the 2,300 false positives they should have. If they had, there would have been minus 730 (1,570 minus 2,300) or in real life data, zero.

The 31st of May 2020 was not unusual. Most days during 2020 saw zero new Covid-19 cases if the 2.3% false positive rate had been deducted from the overall positive test result numbers.

The government never deducted it though. To do so would have bought an end to the "pandemic" overnight. Ergo, the government perpetuated the pandemic – for whatever reason – via the fraudulent manipulation of data. The NHS remained closed down as a result, and patients with cancelled cancer treatment or heart operations died as a direct result of criminal, murderous, governmental fraud.

And it gets worse. British Health Secretary Matt Hancock was confronted about the false positives on live TV by Talk Radio's Julia Hartley-Brewer. Astonishingly, Hancock seemed to be under the impression that the false positive percentage rate should be applied to the positive cases returned, rather than the tests carried out.

If we go back to the PCR tests performed on 21 May 2020 (100,000 tests returning 1,570 positive results) Hancock applied the 2.3% false positive rate to the 1,570 positive results rather than the 100,000 tests.

2.3% of 1,570 equates to 36. So, Hancock subtracted the 36 from the 1,570 and claimed 1,534 true positive test results. As I explained earlier, the true figure was minus 730 (1,570 minus 2,300) or in real life data, zero.

It really shouldn't be possible to drive a tyrannical global pandemic response based on a poor understanding of maths. Hancock should have been sacked on the spot. The pandemic should have ended there and then. It didn't of course.

If there was one thing alone during 2020 which persuaded me that the entire pandemic was a colossal fraud, it was Hancock's dodgy maths (at best) or deliberate malfeasance at worst. The misreading of Covid test data didn't just happen in

Britain of course; the same "mistake" was made across the world.

The sheer enormity - in terms of both tyranny and murderous consequences - of this is almost beyond mere words, but I will write some anyway: a basic "error" was made in establishing the presence of a viral pandemic. Had the error not been made, there would have been no pandemic. The entire political, scientific, medical and journalistic industries failed to notice this most obvious and glaring error....

And it gets worse again. PCR tests are extremely complicated and long-winded. They entail repeated cycles of heating and cooling (in strict laboratory conditions) of the individual test specimens. The standard number of cycles required to determine the existence of a particular viral molecule is 25.

As the number of heating / cooling cycles increases, so too does the chance of creating false positives. The 2.3% false positive average quoted by the government was related to 25 cycles, but when this is upped to 45 cycles the false positive rate rises to 97%.

The government never told us how many cycles were used in the 2020 tests, but it now turns out to have been anywhere between 35 to 45. They were all useless, in other words. The entire thing was a con.

Here are a couple of final thoughts about the PCR testing farce, which might appeal to the more conspiratorial amongst us:

Towards the end of 2020, the government claimed to be processing up to a million PCR tests in a single day. Given the complexity and time involved in each test, one has to wonder if we were being lied to. Does England really have sufficient technicians, laboratories and specialist annealing ovens to carry out such complex tests for a million people daily?

Secondly, why were the nasal swabs so extreme? Why were they rammed so far up our noses? Were they actually designed to harvest something else entirely? Is it possible that the government now holds the DNA record of every single person who was nasally assaulted via a PCR test?

Chapter 9: How It Started

This chapter is a little out of kilter. It should have been chapter one, but I wanted to expose the fraudulent reporting and engineering of purported Covid-19 deaths first. Once everyone understands this criminal fraud, every other fraud relating to Covid-19 falls into place.

We don't know when plans were first hatched to engineer a viral pandemic in 2020. We do know about Event 201 in October 2019 though, which was hosted by Johns Hopkins University and organised by the World Economic Forum and the Bill & Melinda Gates Foundation.

Event 201 centred around a hypothetical global outbreak of a lethal virus and the subsequent response by governments around the world. It laid the groundwork for lockdowns, masking, and social distancing. None of these tyrannical measures had been part of pandemic health policies before. All the centuries-old, tried-and-trusted viral pandemic response plans were torn up and discarded in favour of targeting the healthy, rather than quarantining the ill.

On the whole, people don't want to be locked up at home for the best part of a year and instructed to behave as though they were a lethal danger to all living things. Therefore, they had to be conditioned to obey the New Normal rules and regulations related to Covid-19. In short, they had to be terrorised into compliance.

Enter Neil Ferguson, pandemic modeller extraordinaire of Imperial College London. Ferguson predicted Covid-19 could kill half-a-million people in Britain and two million in America. The international media shrieked these headlines to the world. The politicians gravely warned us we were facing apocalyptic events. The World Health Organisation declared a Global Pandemic. Governments declared national health emergencies. And so began the lockdowns. And so began tyranny.

Neil Ferguson had modelled pandemic scenarios before. In 2005 he predicted two-hundred-million people could die globally from Bird Flu. In reality, only three hundred people died.

In 2009 he predicted sixty-five-thousand deaths in the UK from Swine Flu. Only a few hundred died. In 2002 he predicted up to fifty-thousands deaths in the UK, resulting from eating beef infected with Bovine Spongiform Encephalopathy – otherwise known as Mad Cow Disease. In reality only one hundred and seventy people died.

In 2001 Ferguson's Imperial team produced modelling on foot and mouth disease suggesting animals should be culled without evidence of infection. This led to the slaughter of more than six million perfectly healthy cattle, sheep and pigs.

Hundreds-of-years of selective breeding were wiped out in days. Farmers and their families were reduced to tears and penury. Many experts accused Ferguson of making fundamental errors in the basic data input he shoved into his computer. A subsequent enquiry into Ferguson's report labelled it not fit for purpose.

Yet here he was again in 2020, making his usual The End Is Nigh predictions. How was this possible? How could the predictions of such a ridiculous man with such a tragi-hilarious ability to get everything monumentally wrong, possibly be used to justify the greatest repression of liberty the world had ever seen?

The answer to that is the same answer to so many other questionable Covid-19 lunacies – Bill Gates.

In March 2020, The Bill & Melinda Gates Foundation granted[1] Imperial College London (Neil Ferguson's employer) an eye-watering seventy-nine million dollars. Sums of money this huge effectively buy whatever outcome the financier wants.

If the financier also provides multi-million-dollar grants to the mainstream global media (which Bill Gates does) he can then broadcast it to the world without any irritating questions from independent journalists, such as "is Neil Ferguson a trustworthy sort of a chap we should listen to with due reverence on matters of supreme importance?"

Of course he is not, and of course he was not. He was bought and paid for. His terror-porn death predictions were simply used to generate fear and hysteria around the world. This was particularly useful in forcing the hand of politicians. Yes, they could ignore the lunatic predictions of this ridiculous man, but suppose they came true? Suppose millions actually died? That would be the end of their political careers. Far safer then, career-wise, to lockdown the healthy in an unprecedented act of tyranny. Which they duly did.

What is even worse in this tawdry tale of purchased tyranny, is that some decent and honest scientists did what the presstitute journalists refused to do – they demanded to see Ferguson's Covid Catastophe arithmetic.

Ferguson initially stated a lot of it was in his head and had not been recorded. When he finally handed it over for closer inspection, it was torn to shreds. Accusations of "garbage data" fed into the modelling computer came thick and fast. Nonetheless, the accusers were ignored, and Bill Gates got the global emergency he had paid for.

Chapter 10: Lockdowns

Lockdown was never referred to as "lockdown" in March 2020. We were "asked" to stay at home for a few weeks, thus allowing our health services to get up to speed without being swamped. As we now know, a few weeks became months became 2021.

I simply cannot believe this was not planned. The logistics involved in keeping a country afloat after closing down the economy are extremely complicated. Months - if not years - of planning must have gone into this.

One of the strangest things about the first lockdown in the UK was the enforcement date of March the 26th, just one week after the government declared on March 19th that Covid-19 was being downgraded from a High Consequence Infectious Disease (HCID). The reason given for the downgrade was a low mortality rate......

Anyway, the world locked down. When it became apparent the lockdowns were going to stay in place until a miracle vaccine was discovered, the governments promised us detailed cost/benefit analyses would be conducted. They never were. But they very much should have been.

The principal reason they should, is all to do with deaths. Closing down the country also meant partially closing down health services to non-Covid patients. Inculcating fear meant many people were too scared to go anywhere near a hospital. Patients with cancer and heart problems stayed away - voluntarily or involuntarily. Many of them died as a result.

On the 19th of July 2020, the Daily Telegraph published[1] an article based on Office for National Statistics figures, claiming two-hundred-thousand people could die (mid to long term) in the UK due to lockdowns. Similar figures were published in countries all around the world.

Here is a brutal truth. Governments which locked down, essentially stated the following: "We are going to murder XYZ thousand people. We undertake this crime because we *think* we might save other people from Covid-19 deaths."

Even more remarkably, the death rates were completely normal before lockdowns were initiated. Lockdowns were not the forced result of having to deal with large numbers of deaths. Rather, large numbers of deaths were the forced result of government instructed lockdowns. It is difficult to understand quite why our politicians are not locked up for life after successful prosecution for Crimes Against Humanity.

Worse again, lockdowns enabled the Great Care Home Cull. Which means the government locked us down in the full knowledge this would kill people, and then utilised the lockdown to kill even more people in the care homes. It really is no exaggeration to talk about Crimes Against Humanity.

And it was all so unnecessary. Covid-19 presented no statistical noteworthy threat of death to the healthy – of any age. All the data between January 2020 and December 2023 (when this is being written) supports this statement. It is not a claim. It is not an opinion. It is a data-verifiable fact.

There was a world of lockdown difference between middle-class families and working-class families. Large houses with gardens afforded relaxation and contentment for the middle-class, especially so with monthly furlough scheme deposits pinging into their bank accounts on the first of every month.

The working-class were nowhere near as fortunate. Many found themselves unable to satisfy the government's furlough scheme conditions and were rendered destitute as a result. Many lived in cramped flats without gardens. If they tried to escape for a walk in the local park, they encountered violently hostile policemen who were "only following orders".

The consequences of lockdowns are all around us. Health services have fragmented. Waiting times are through the roof. Once treatable cancer and heart patients are dying before they can be treated. Suicides are up. Mental health problems are up. Educational standards have plummeted. Truancy rates have soared. Tens-of thousands of children have disappeared from school completely. Bankruptcies are rising. Child abuse soared during lockdown.

Conclusion: Lockdowns caused inevitable deaths. They enabled tens-of-thousands of "deaths" in the care homes we were unable to visit. Lockdowns saved no deaths because Covid-19 lacked sufficient lethality to kill anyone without one foot already in the grave. Lockdowns caused social, financial, and emotional misery for the most vulnerable. Lockdowns bankrupted nations whilst enriching the Western elites. They also caused huge numbers of death in the developing world, where children starved to death because the governments didn't have the financial luxury of paying workers not to work. Truly, lockdowns were a veritable Crime Against Humanity.

Chapter 11: Did Lockdowns, Masks & Social Distancing Work?

Lockdowns: No, lockdowns didn't work. This is simply because there was never such a thing as total lockdown, where every single person remained holed up in their property for months on end. Even if this had happened, it would have had no effect whatsoever on a virus transported in the air we breathe, and in the air all around us all of the time.

It seems to be some kind of middle-class fantasy that the outside world stopped turning in late March 2020. Whilst Charles and Arabella (both BBC executives) hunkered down for the duration, the electrical supply powering their Netflix binge-watching remained in perfect operation, courtesy of horny handed men shinning up pylons.

Trinkets were delivered to their door by heavily accented men in vans. Food miraculously appeared on their local Waitrose shelves. Whatever their little hearts desired could by magicked up at the click of an iPhone button, after which the working-class scuttled and scurried their errands in a supposedly viral soup to ensure the middle-class enjoyed a lockdown life of relaxed contentment.

Above the middle-class came the political class who, as we now know, partied hard and partied often. And above them came the billionaire class, who jetted around the world whenever and wherever they wanted. It was really only the middle-class who salaciously locked down and narcissistically assumed the rest of the world locked down with them.

The most glaring example of the whole lockdown hypocrisy/uselessness could be found in the realm of supermarkets, where workers toiled away for the entirety of lockdown. Pretty much everyone went to a supermarket. Those who didn't, simply took advantage of home delivery via a man in a van who, of course, mixed with lots of people between supermarket pick-up to home delivery in upmarket suburbia.

Supermarket workers in the Western world were exposed to 80% plus of all local humanity thronging their stores. Supermarket workers were the ultimate Disease Control Group. Did thousands of them keel over and die from Covid-19? No, they did not. Did thousands of them become very ill? No, they did not.

Unlike the lockdowners, supermarket workers got plenty of exercise, sunshine and fresh air, all of which provide a good defence against viruses. As do Vitamins C/D and zinc. We were never told to make sure we had sufficient vitamins though. Instead, we were told to avoid exercise, sunshine and fresh air. This obvious and medically criminal lunacy should have set alarm bells ringing from the outset.

Conclusion. Lockdowns could never have worked anyway, courtesy of the capability of an airborne virus to get anywhere and everywhere. Lockdowns were completely unnecessary, as evidenced by the good health of supermarket workers exposed for months on end to the massed ranks of humanity. Finally, lockdowns weren't even lockdowns, due to the servant class frantically dashing about in attendance to the privileged class.

Something else to bear in mind is the importance of isolation when it comes to brainwashing. In the 1970s, Russia's KGB security service carried out psychological experiments on captive civilians held in solitary confinement isolation. The results suggested that when someone was isolated and bombarded with propaganda designed to instil fear, it took just 66 days to bring about a state of mind closed to facts, reason and logic, but open to any misinformation promising to alleviate the fear, no matter how fantastical.

Our purportedly benign political elite has adopted similar KGB tactics in the purportedly free and democratic West, resulting in the herd insanity we saw around us in 2020. The fanatical mask wearers, social distancers and experimental vaccine believers, all conditioned by continual 24/7 propaganda coupled with lockdown isolation techniques previously conducted only in horror-show dictatorships.

Masks: If you Google "peer reviewed studies masks Covid-19" you will find approximately one gazillion highly referenced articles penned by gimlet-glass wearing scientists peering short-sightedly through expensive microscopes. All of their studies are useless. In a non-Sovietesque world, they would have been laughed out of peer-reviewed court.

The reason is very simple. The Covid-19 virus is many times smaller than the gaps in the mesh of the most expensive and tightly woven face masks, let alone the cheap ones. This is why scientists working with dangerous pathogens/viruses in laboratories wear astronaut style suits and helmets with an independent air-supply.

It is why firemen wear sealed breathing apparatus to avoid smoke inhalation. Smoke molecules, by the way, are ten-times larger than the Covid-19 Virus. It is why paint-sprayers in car repair body shops wear sealed masks with an independent air supply.

Wearing a bit of cheap cloth round your chops in the hope it will stop a virus is no more ridiculously futile than attempting to snare plankton in a heavy-duty rope fishing net designed to catch ten-kilo Cod, or whacking great Groupers.

Masks do have two particularly useful attributes though. The first is that they signify, very easily and obviously, our level of compliance. Do not for one moment think government agents were not wandering the streets and supermarkets, carefully noting the numbers wearing or not wearing masks, before reporting back the latest "Compliance Indicator" to their political bosses.

The second useful attribute is that they make people ill, thus causing more fear in the community. Damp, warm, unwashed bits of cloth across your mouth and nose are ideal breeding grounds for bacteria, which are then sucked straight into your lungs. One wonders how many mask wearers went on to suffer from bacterial pneumonia during the viral pandemic which should, as the name suggests, have caused only viral pneumonia.

Social Distancing: There is really nothing to say about this. One can only assume the enforcement of it appealed to some demonic sense of humour prevalent within our political class. Air moves around. The Covid-19 virus is transported in the air. Keeping a precise two metres from Granny in her kitchen no more protects her from an airborne virus than hoping her feet will remain dry provided we keep a sufficient distance from Granny whilst paddling in the sea.

As I say, the whole social distancing lunacy must surely have been a demonic joke. Who says politicians don't have a sense of humour?

Conclusion: Control. It was all about and only about control. Lockdowns, masks, and social distancing were simply tyrannical theatre, designed to create fear, compliance visibility, illness, and a conditioned submissive response to political edicts. It was very powerful. Some of us refused to wear masks, but it took a degree of courage to do so, particularly for the first time.

The last four years have something of a dreamlike quality to them. It is still hard to accept what has been done to 99.99 percent of the population by a handful of criminals within the political, medical, media, and scientific industrial complex. But there can be no argument about the terrible sins they have committed. Their evil is contained within the facts and figures on their very own data gathering sites.

2020 was a global crime scene. There is no other way of describing it. The greatest crime came later though, in the coerced vaccination of a brainwashed and bamboozled population with a needless gene engineering potion as dangerous as it is useless. Everything about Covid-19 vaccines revolves around crime and fraud. And everything on Planet Covid orbits a malignant white dwarf and an ever-expanding black hole sucking all that is good and honest and decent into cosmic oblivion via the Gates of Hell.

Chapter 12: Do I Need the Covid Vaccine?

Governments all around the world displayed an astonishing degree of fanaticism with regard to vaccinating everyone against Covid-19. It was truly mind-boggling to both watch and be part of. Despite the millions of argumentative words generated between pro-vax hysterics and anti-vax sceptics, there are really only three simple questions to be asked about the Covid vaccine:

Do I need it? Does it work? Is it safe?

Do I need it?

As I have outlined earlier, there was no lethal pandemic in 2020. The Infection Fatality Rate for Covid-19 was similar to that of influenza, so nobody needed an experimental, Emergency Use Authorisation vaccine at all, let alone the young, healthy, or pregnant.

Somewhat ironically, this was revealed in the drug trials themselves. AstraZeneca stated they "were running out of time" with regard to their vaccine trial and went on to explain this was because they were having great trouble finding anyone who exhibited Covid-19 symptoms, which obviously caused data input problems when it came to comparisons between the vaccinated and unvaccinated trial members.

The Pfizer vaccine trial consisted of 42,000 people, but only 170 of them (0.4%) tested positive for Covid-19. Of these 170 people, none became seriously ill or needed hospitalisation. Interestingly enough though, there were a handful of hospitalisations, but these were only amongst the vaccinated trial members whose health problems were caused by the vaccine side effects rather than Covid-19.

What the Pfizer trial inadvertently revealed was obvious; Covid-19 was nothing to worry about. Hardly anyone contracted it and of those that did, no one was badly affected by it. The vaccine was therefore unnecessary at best, and at worst was responsible for severe side-effects and hospitalisations. The whole Covid farce should have been called to a halt there and then, but that didn't happen of course.

Chapter 13: Does it work?

No, the Covid-19 vaccines are not effective at all. They don't stop infection or transmission, contrary to what we were told at the time. When it became apparent they didn't do what a vaccine is supposed to do (stop infection and transmission) we were then told the vaccine was effective in minimising the infection and keeping us out of hospital.

This was a lie. No one actually knew if this was the case. Nothing in the vaccine trial suggested this might be true and, more to the point, the claimed minimisation of infection was never actually tested or evaluated in any of the trials. As I say, this was simply a lie.

Do you remember the fanfare in late 2020 when we were told vaccine redemption was close to hand? Do you remember the adulation and the frenzied gratitude toward those lovely, thoughtful, deeply caring people in the Big Pharma Industry who arrived like the heroic cavalry at the 11th hour to save us all from certain death?

The vaccine is 95% effective we were told. Hoorah for the vaccine! And out most of us duly trudged to wait in line for our jab of salvation. What did they mean by 95% effective though? Effective against what, exactly? If the vaccines didn't stop infection, transmission, severity of illness or death, where on earth did the "effective" in 95% effective come from?

We were led to believe it simply meant that out of every one-hundred vaccinated people, ninety-five could happily get Covid-19 and shake it off in a jiffy, whilst five unfortunate people would not. This is not the case at all, though, and has to do with Absolute Risk Reduction (ARR) and Relative Risk Reduction (RRR).

Approximately forty-two thousand people were involved in the Pfizer vaccine trial. Twenty-one thousand were given the vaccine, and twenty-one thousand a placebo. The latter is known as the Control Group. A few weeks later both groups were tested for signs of Covid-19 symptoms such as a cough, cold, fever etc, which were "confirmed" by a positive PCR test.

In the vaccinated group, eight cases of Covid-19 were discovered, and in the control group, one hundred and sixty-two. Eight is 5% of one hundred and sixty-two, which allowed Pfizer to claim a 95% effectiveness RRR rate (If only 5% of the vaccinated tested positive, it presumes a 95% efficacy rate *relative* to the unvaccinated).

This means nothing of course, considering less than 1% of the unvaccinated control group contracted Covid-19. An RRR of 95% in no way suggests the vaccine is 95% efficient in stopping an infection. It is basically an accountancy sleight-of-hand. It is a real-world medical fraud.

You will notice the numbers of those infected were extremely small. This presented a marketing problem for Pfizer. Only 0.4% of the 42,000 people involved in the trial tested positive for Covid-19. This effectively means 99.6% of them were at no risk from Covid-19 regardless of vaccination or not.

I won't bore you with the maths, but this leads to an Absolute Risk Reduction (ARR) of just 0.86% which is not terribly useful when it comes to selling a vaccine to the public. A 95% RRR efficacy sounds so much better than a 0.86% ARR efficacy, doesn't it?

 In normal times, both the ARR and RRR percentages are clearly stated with regard to a vaccine. But not in 2020, the year of lies and fraud on a colossal scale. Refusing to divulge the weedy 0.86% ARR (whilst pretending the 95% RRR meant a real-world 95% effectiveness in stopping an infection) may have only been a lie via omission, but in terms of scale it was a veritable whopper.

Chapter 14: Is It Safe?

No, the Covid vaccines are not safe. Before I get into this though, here is a quote from George Orwell's dystopian novel *1984*: "*The Party told you to reject the evidence of your eyes and ears. It was their final, most essential command.*"

Why do I mention this? Because I cannot ignore what I have seen and heard about the vaccines. My social group is not particularly large; friends and friends of friends probably amount to no more than a couple of hundred people. Yet within this relatively small circle I know of two deaths post-vaccine, one of them a professional cyclist in his thirties.

I know of three instances of myocarditis in young men, and several other heart related issues. Every Saturday and Sunday morning I used to hear the thwacking footsteps of a fifty-something chap called Matt as he ran past my bedroom window. Matt doesn't run anymore. He is now confined to a wheelchair.

As for blood clots and thrombotic issues, I know of at least five. Prior to 2021 I didn't know anyone suddenly falling foul of these problems. Nor did I know, in 2020, of a single person who became ill or even a but sniffily from Covid-19. As I say then, I cannot ignore the evidence of my eyes and ears.

This is anecdotal, obviously, but is it borne out by official data? Yes, it is. Vaccine injury databases in Britain, Europe and America suggest that in just three years there have been more deaths, maiming's, serious injuries and minor injuries caused by the Covid-19 vaccines than all the other non-Covid vaccines **combined** over the last thirty years.

See the following graphs:

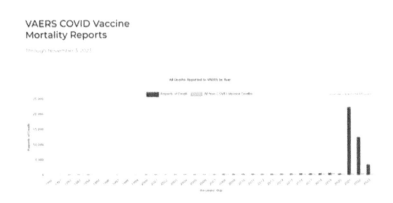

Source of graph[1]

VAERS COVID Vaccine
Permanently Disabled Reports

Through November 1, 2023

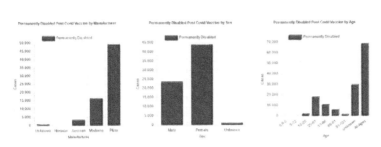

Source of graph[2]

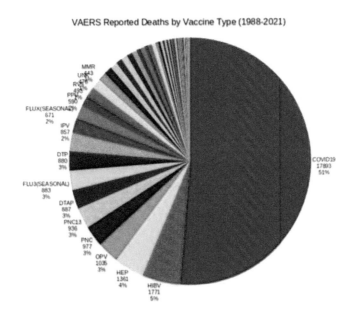

VAERS Reported Deaths by Vaccine Type (1988-2021)

In early 2023, Pfizer CEO Albert Bourla was interviewed by CNBC in Davos. The journalist seemed to be aware of vaccine injuries and nervously pressed him – very lightly – as to whether the Pfizer booster was causing heart attacks, strokes etc. Bourla replied thus:

"The CDC (Centres for Disease Control and Prevention) triggered a comprehensive review of all databases in existence, and they discovered nothing. The same is with us (Pfizer)… we found nothing, not a single safety signal although we have distributed billions of doses."

Pfizer CEO Albert Bourla is a liar. Quite apart from the horrifying VAERS figures above, which Bourla is only too well aware of, Pfizer's own documentation[3] (which they were legally forced to release in May 2021) states the following:

"Pfizer has also taken multiple actions to help alleviate the large increase of adverse event reports. This includes significant technology enhancements as well as increasing the number of data entry and case processing colleagues."

The adverse events consisted of 42,086 cases, out of which a disproportionate number were female (29,914). Age was also disproportionate, with the largest majority coming within the 31 to 50-year-old demographic.

Their adverse side-effects were not trivial. For example, there were 25,957 nervous system disorders. 17,283 Musculo-skeletal and connective tissue disorders. 14,096 gastro-intestinal disorders and 8,476 skin and subcutaneous tissue disorders.

There were also 1,223 deaths. These figures are as shocking as they are astonishing. It should be noted they all occurred before the end of February 2021. The vaccine roll-out only started in December 2020, so it is just two months of data really – if that.

Is it a coincidence that excess deaths and permanent disabilities are up in all the countries with high vaccination rates? This has been the case over 2021, 2022 and 2023. Indeed, the higher the vaccine take-up, the higher the percentage of excess deaths. Many countries are seeing similar excess deaths – and higher – than the pandemic year of 2020. Yet the politicians and media refuse to recognise this disastrous situation, let alone talk about it.

One can hardly blame them of course. Their policies, enforced through coercion, are completely to blame. If they recognised the consequences of their actions, then they open themselves up to criminal prosecution for their actions. They will never allow this, of course, because we are quite literally talking about Democide here.

There is one particular and unarguable reality which suggests the vaccines are directly linked to excess deaths, and it is that of Africa and other poorer countries which could not afford mass vaccinations. Western doctors and scientists are baffled, apparently, about the normal levels of deaths seen in Africa during Pandemic 2020, and the normal level of deaths between 2021-2024 which saw a fraction of the vaccination rates compared to the West.

Africa has very few Care Homes, which explains the normal death rates in 2020. Africa had very low vaccination rates, which explains the normal death rates between 2021 and 2024. Myopic doctors and scientists with bulging bank accounts remain "baffled" as to why this might be. Sherlock Holmes wouldn't be baffled at all.

Conclusion: We didn't need the vaccines. And I think it is fair to say that in terms of efficacy and safety, the vaccines are as useless as they are dangerous. The whole Covid-19 vaccine issue is a gigantic, murderous fraud. Worse, it is a gigantic murderous fraud built on the earlier gigantic murderous fraud of an alleged Covid-19 pandemic. Perhaps now is a good time to remind our utterly corrupt politicians and utterly corrupt members of the medical and pharmaceutical industry what the exact definition of Democide is:

"The killing of members of a country's civilian population as a result of its government's policy, including by direct action, indifference, and neglect."

Chapter 15: The Pfizer Trial

Whilst the world was avidly watching the Pfizer vaccine trial hoping to hear the vaccines were safe and would thus save mankind from dying out, a much more important issue became glaringly obvious – which is that the vaccine trials themselves were completely unnecessary, and possibly riddled with fraud.

Pfizer's PR blurb[1] regarding its Covid-19 vaccine trial opens with the following sentence: "*The Phase 3 clinical trial was designed to determine if the Pfizer-BioNTech COVID-19 vaccine is safe and effective in preventing COVID-19 disease.*"

Did the trial determine if the vaccine was safe and effective in preventing Covid-19 disease? No, it actually proved the exact opposite. It was as ineffective as it was dangerous. It failed all three of its stated endpoints. It should never have been authorised. The fact that it was is testament to the lies and crimes committed post 2020. And it gets worse:

Pfizer "lost" ninety-two people from their forty-two thousand people vaccine trial. This is a relatively low number, but it becomes supremely important considering Pfizer's 95% Relative Risk Rate (RRR) efficacy was based on only eight people from the vaccinated cohort testing positive for Covid-19, compared to the one hundred and sixty-two in the unvaccinated cohort.

Suppose though, the ninety-two people "lost" by Pfizer were lost because they were vaccinated AND tested positive for Covid-19? If this was the case, and had they been included, Pfizer's claimed 95% RRR would have dropped to just a 39% RRR efficacy rate, and the trial would have been declared a failure.

Theoretically speaking, it might be even worse than I have described. When forty-two thousand people are observed over six-months, it is quite normal for some of them to die. In this instance, thirty-eight did just that, split roughly 50:50 between vaccinated and unvaccinated. Some experts have stated their surprise at just thirty-eight deaths out of forty-two thousand. A more usual number, they say, would be at least one hundred.

Is it possible the ninety-two people "lost" by Pfizer were vaccinated and died from adverse side effects? Were they deliberately lost because to admit what had happened meant kissing goodbye to tens-of-billions of dollars in government sponsored mass vaccine sales?

A decent, moral and ethical company would not, **could not** behave in such a manner, obviously, but is Pfizer a decent, moral and ethical company? I would say emphatically not, as I will explain.

Chapter 16: Pfizer's Criminal Past.

As we have seen, Pfizer CEO Albert Bourla flat out lied about safety signals regarding the Covid-19 vaccine. Does he have previous form for dishonesty? That we don't yet know, but does Pfizer itself have a history of dishonesty, fraud and multiple deaths linked to its products? You bet it does.

Between 2000 to 2020, Pfizer was involved in multiple lawsuits and made multiple payouts to the tune of an astonishing $4.7 billion dollars. In long hand, that is 470,000,000,000 dollars.

The list of claims against Pfizer related to the following: manipulating drug trials, bribery of officials, causing deaths and disabilities, lying about deaths and disabilities, falsifying data, violating federal anti-racketeering laws etc. Over a billion dollars was paid out for offences related to dodgy government contracts. Hello, Ursula von der Leyen and many others!

In November 2021, the *British Medical Journal*[1] revealed the *Ventavia Research Group* (sub-contracted by Pfizer) had falsified data, unblinded patients, employed inadequately trained vaccinators, and was slow to follow up on adverse events reported in the crucial phase III trial for Pfizer's COVID-19 vaccine.

I rather think this answers my earlier question then, regarding the moral and ethical virtue of Pfizer prohibiting it from lying about the missing ninety-two people in the vaccine trial. Pfizer clearly lies all of the time when billions of dollars are involved. There is every reason to believe they lied about the missing people in the Covid vax trial, considering the vast sales due in 2021 (and onwards) dwarfed anything Pfizer had ever achieved before.

Conclusion: I am going to quote Simon Elmer here. Simon has forensically researched everything Covid-19 related, and elegantly and concisely written it up in his book *The Road to Fascism: For a Critique of the Global Biosecurity State*[2] which I highly recommend. His words then, are my conclusion. They are simply too good not to be pinched and used here:

"Given this record of ongoing corruption and malpractice from which only its enormous profits, political influence and systemic bribery of officials have saved it from criminal prosecution, it seems extraordinary that Pfizer is still permitted to manufacture and sell any health care products. Yet this is the pharmaceutical company we're being asked by the UK Government to trust with the mass vaccination of 68 million people via a product that has been rushed through clinical trials in 7 months, using an experimental technology that has never before been approved and whose side effects are still

*unknown, for a disease with the fatality rate of
seasonal influenza, which statistically is a threat only
to those over 70 years old with serious pre-existing
medical conditions, and for which there is no evidence
that it prevents infection by a virus for which only 1%
of the population is currently testing positive with a
testing programme that has an average false positive
rate higher than the number of positive cases
reported."*

Chapter 17: Is It Even a Vaccine?

The Covid-19 mRNA vaccines are an entirely new and experimental means of combating disease. Vaccines in the past were simply a weakened – and thus safe - version of a dangerous virus. When Injected into the body they safely kick-started the immune system into building a defence against the full-strength virus capable of seriously damaging or killing humans.

The new Covid-19 vaccines don't do this. They contain a genetic sequencing code which instructs our body to create spike proteins. The immune system recognises the manufactured spike proteins as dangerous and initiates its natural resistance operation.

The spike proteins are not the virus, but they are dangerous because they provide (and were designed in a laboratory to provide) the mechanism which allows a virus to enter our cells. The truly bizarre aspect of this is that during 2020 we were locked down, muzzled and terrorised for one reason only – which was to avoid contracting the spike protein present in the Covid-19 virus.

And then, in late 2020 and throughout 2021, we were fanatically encouraged and coerced into taking a vaccine specifically designed to carry out one single task, which was to instruct our own bodies to manufacture the exact same spike protein we had been "encouraged" to avoid contracting in 2020. This really should make people extraordinarily angry........

We were (and still are) told the vaccine-induced manufacturing of spike proteins in our bodies would only last for a few days, but that appears to be yet another criminal lie. Many people who accepted the vaccines now find themselves repeatedly suffering from colds, coughs, influenza and chronic fatigue.

The term "Long Covid" is propagandised as long-term ill-effects resulting from contracting Covid-19, but it is much more likely that the vaccine-induced spike proteins, which allow viruses to enter our cells, continue to be manufactured in the bodies of mRNA vaccinated people and are thus opening the cellular-level door to every single respiratory virus currently doing the rounds.

This is much the same as AIDS or Acquired Immune Deficiency Syndrome. AIDS didn't kill humans; it simply lowered the ability of our immune systems to counter-act viruses that could. If the Covid-19 vaccines continue to instruct our bodies to manufacture spike proteins, then all the people who took them might just as well have been jabbed with a serum containing AIDS.

I mentioned earlier that the vaccines contain a genetic sequencing code. Many people are still unaware that this code is manufactured by a computer and is the exact same code first developed to manufacture the Covid-19 virus in China's Wuhan Institute of Virology. This, again, is something people should be extraordinarily angry about.

Just as they should be about the genetic aspect of these crimes. mRNA vaccines are gene-therapy, which your doctor, health regulatory agency, President/Prime Minister **never** informed you about. Nonetheless, that is precisely what they are, and we see them doled out to babies, toddlers, pregnant women and healthy people of all ages.

An article[1] in the *Daily Telegraph* (6 December 2023) discusses problems with this genetic platform: "mRNA jabs, such as the ones created by Moderna and Pfizer, use a string of genetic material to tell the body to create a specific protein.... and that problems arise when the genetic sequence is misread - which leads to 'frame-shifting' and the production of rogue proteins which can lead to immune system flare-ups."

One of the "experts" the DT quoted was Professor Anne Willis, Director of Cambridge University's Medical Research Council (MRC) Toxicology Unit. She admitted there were genetic sequencing problems with Covid-19 mRNA vaccines which caused an astonishing 1 in 4 people injected with the Pfizer/Moderna genetic sequencing serums to experience an unintended immunity response.

Such a horrifying admission didn't seem to unduly concern Prof Willis though. She is, according to the DT: "very excited that there is a way to fix this issue, which massively de-risks this platform (mRNA) going-forward."

I'm sure we are all terribly reassured to hear this, but it might have been better to sort it out before injecting billions of people with it, no? And what are we to make of the blithe dismissal of immune system flare-ups? From what I can gather, such events can be life threatening.

Normal vaccines take at least ten years to produce, such is the complexity of drug trials. A mere handful of people experiencing death or serious injury as a vaccine side effect would be sufficient to cancel the trial and pull the drug.

mRNA vaccines are not normal vaccines. They are not, in reality, vaccines at all. They are a form of human genetic modification. As such they are subject to much more stringent drug trials and should take a great deal longer than the normal ten years for non-genetic drugs. This was thrown out of the window in 2020.

The refusal to honestly label them as a gene-based therapy enabled our governments to inject us with them after just a few months of trials. Our politicians lied to us, as did Pfizer and Moderna. Most shockingly - and criminally - every single one of our health regulatory agencies, whose sole remit is to protect the health of a country's citizens, lied to us as well.

All lies. All crime.

Chapter 18. Rewriting Medical Language

In order to facilitate the Covid-19 pandemic, a rewriting of medical language was necessary. Prior to 2020 the term "pandemic" described a global health emergency with large numbers of deaths.

Post 2020, this was changed to simply describing a health situation with many infections, or cases, rather than deaths.

The term "herd immunity" once used as an expression describing natural immunity developed by massed humanity's exposure to an infection, was changed to a health situation made possible only by massed vaccination.

Even the term "vaccine" was changed. Prior to 2020 it described a pharmaceutical which **prevented** an infectious disease. Post 2020 this was changed to a pharmaceutical which merely provided **protection** against an infectious disease.

The level of "protection" was not detailed. All this rewriting should have caused alarm bells to ring amongst politicians, scientists, and journalists. Sadly though, it did no such thing.

Chapter 19: Afterword.

The sole purpose of this small book was to show, in as few words as possible, that there was no lethal Covid-19 pandemic in 2020, and that the vaccines were completely unnecessary, horrifically dangerous in some cases, and astonishingly / criminally ineffective in every possible way a vaccine is supposed to be effective.

There is so much more to say about this crime of the century, but to do so would require much more than one book. The roles played by Bill Gates and Anthony Fauci, for example, could fill an entire bookshelf.

The details laid out in this book are not just my opinion; they are taken from data sites owned by governments and health regulation agencies. They are true. And if they are true, then everything we were told (and continue to be told) about Covid-19 is a lie.

Tragically – and criminally – the people lying to us are those whose specific job it is to look after our best interests. The politicians, the doctors, the health regulatory agencies, the mainstream media, the Fact Check agencies, the World Health Organisation, the EU, the UN, and the social media giants such as Facebook and YouTube.

All of these people and organisations amassed money and power during the Covid-19 purported pandemic. This money and power resulted purely from lying to and betraying the citizens of nations worldwide.

In America, the Food & Drug Agency (FDA) only released Pfizer's data on vaccine harms because it was forced to do so by a court order. Also in America, The Centers for Disease Control and Prevention (CDC) continues to recommend pregnant women and babies receive mRNA booster shots, whilst simultaneously fighting court cases to prevent the release of data they hold which catalogues massive numbers of vaccine harms.

The same thing is happening in every single Western country, where every single health regulation agency is doing the exact same thing. The levels of corruption are vast. As are the wicked and murderous crimes they are engaged in. The CDC's motto, incidentally, is: *Saving Lives. Protecting People.*

Hundreds-of-thousands of people, possibly millions, have died as a result of the wall-to-wall lies and corruption. It is my fervent hope that one day all those responsible will stand trial for having committed crimes against humanity. This seems unlikely, given the power and control they currently exert, but we must never give up.

Even if we never see Fauci, Gates, Bourla, Biden, Ardern, Daniel Andrews, Whitty, Walensky etc in court, we can at least let them know that **we know** what they did; that we know they are criminals no different and no better than the 20th century leaders of the Nazi and Communist regimes who also committed crimes against humanity.

Finally, and I'm pretty sure many of you are aware of this, *they* are going to try to do it again. Probably this year. Be prepared and be brave. If they are not halted, our future will be that of slaves living under a New World Order Tyranny enforced by Digital ID, Electronic Vaccine Passports and government-controlled bank accounts courtesy of Central Bank Digital Currency. I firmly believe a future bio-fascist digital tyranny is what the Covid-19 "pandemic" was all about and only about from the get-go.

References

Chapter 2. Fraudulent Excess Deaths

1: https://tinyurl.com/3jya9enb

Chapter 3: Manufacturing Excess Deaths

1: https://tinyurl.com/y8pnse8w

Chapter 5: Matt Hancock's Role

1: https://tinyurl.com/43642jcb

2: https://tinyurl.com/32twxe6p

3: https://tinyurl.com/y3k4yksm

4: https://tinyurl.com/ycy4cp66

5: https://tinyurl.com/38a55bw2

6: https://tinyurl.com/mry27s2y

Chapter 7: Flu Deaths V Covid-19 Deaths in 2020

1: https://tinyurl.com/4745h8hb

2: https://tinyurl.com/27crmb7d

3: https://tinyurl.com/27crmb7d

4: https://tinyurl.com/57djrxsk

Chapter 8: The PCR Fraud

1: https://tinyurl.com/mryuc7fc

2: https://tinyurl.com/bdh6m2hh

Chapter 9: How It Started

1: https://tinyurl.com/56n5tzem

Chapter 10: Lockdowns

1: https://tinyurl.com/bdctavp2

Chapter 14: Is It Safe?

1: https://openvaers.com/covid-data/mortality

2: https://openvaers.com/covid-data/disabled

3: https://tinyurl.com/mrxjzffr

Chapter 15: The Pfizer Trial

1: https://tinyurl.com/mvd8drzx

Chapter 16: Pfizer's Criminal Past

1: https://tinyurl.com/mt7bp9z7

2: https://tinyurl.com/ttz67jm9

Chapter 17: Is It Even a Vaccine?

1: https://tinyurl.com/4ptw9cf8

Printed in Great Britain
by Amazon

46494756R00066